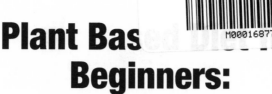

Plant Based Diet for Beginners:

4 week program for an easy transition to a healthy, fit and energetic body

Table of content:

Introduction

I want to thank you and congratulate you for purchasing the book, Plant Based Diet for Beginners: *4 week program to an easy transition to a healthy, fit and energetic body.*

In this book, which is a beginners' guide for transitioning to a completely plant based diet, you are going to learn the benefits of such eating habits and why you should start introducing changes to your meal plan today. Most importantly, you are going to learn how to make this transition easily and effortlessly by following this 4 week program, which includes healthy and delicious recipes for you to try out. The program is designed to help you transition to a plant based diet gradually, thus reducing your cravings for products you are trying to avoid. By following this 4 week transition plan, you will be able to completely switch to a plant based diet and enjoy a better and healthier life.

A plant based diet is a healthy diet in which one does not consume animal products. Instead, one consumes food such as vegetables, fruits, whole grains, beans and nuts. Following a plant based diet means excluding meat and all kinds of animal products from your diet, which are associated with many diseases such as strokes, diabetes, cardiovascular diseases and colon cancer. Thus, transitioning to a plant based diet is going to have plenty of benefits for your physical health, and your mental health as well. Thanks to a lot of fiber, vitamins and other nutrients you are going to be taking in through a plant based diet, you are going to stay energetic and productive throughout the day without ever wanting to go back to your old eating habits!

Chapter 1: What We are Supposed to be Eating According to Human Anatomy

With tons of diet and nutrition plans available today it is safe to say that we as humans have lost track of what are the right foods for our health. The best way to get back on track in terms of our eating habits is to look at the anatomy chart and stick to the foods we were best designed to eat. To do so, you must be familiar with all vertebrates and the differences between their body types.

The word "vertebrate" comes from "vertebrae", which are the bones that make up the spine. Thus, "vertebrate" is used to describe animals that possess a spinal cord surrounded by bone or cartilage. Vertebrates include birds, fish, reptiles and mammals. Therefore, we, humans, fold under this category as well. If we were to compare the anatomy of each vertebrate to one another, we would find significant differences in body types, which determine the psychological food of the species.

There are four groups of vertebrates, including carnivore, omnivore, herbivore and frugivore. Carnivores eat the meat of other animals, omnivores eat both meat of other animals and plants, herbivores eat only plants while frugivores are fruit eaters, including fruits, vegetables and nuts. Most humans sort themselves under the category of omnivores, that is, eaters of both meat and plants. However, when it comes to anatomy, the human anatomy is much closer to that of a frugivore. Let's compare these vertebrate body types to see the difference.

Carnivore

— Examples of carnivore species include cheetah, leopard, lion, jaguar, etc.

— The psychological food of these animals is meat.

— These animals walk on four paws with sharply developed claws.

— Their mouth opening is large, with teeth structure consisting of short and pointed incisors, great sharp fangs and blade shaped molars.

— These animals shear and rip apart their food and swallow it without chewing.

— They have small salivary glands and their acid saliva contains no ptyalin.

— Carnivore species possess a strong hydrochloric acid and they don't require fiber to stimulate peristalsis.

— These animals metabolize large amounts of vitamin A and cholesterol.

— Their sweat glands are located in their paws, while in order to cool their blood they gasp.

— The intestine of Carnivore animals is 1.5 to 3 times of their spine length.

— Their colon is short and contains smooth alkaline.

— These animals complete their digestion process within 2 to 4 hours and they are not able to metabolize cellulose.

Omnivore

— Examples of omnivore species include pigs, bears, chickens, foxes, hedgehogs, etc.

— The psychological food of the omnivore species includes both meat and plants.

— Just like the carnivore species, the omnivore ones have a large mouth opening with a specific teeth structure including sharp fangs, short and pointed incisors, and blade shaped molars.

— They eat their food by shearing it and swallowing it without chewing.

— Their salivary glands are small and their acid saliva contains no ptyalin.

— These animals also have a strong hydrochloric acid and don't require fiber to stimulate peristalsis.

— Similar to carnivores, omnivore species metabolize large amounts of vitamin A and cholesterol.

— Their sweat glands are structured throughout their whole body.

— The intestine of omnivore animals is 10 times their spine length.

— These animals cannot metabolize cellulose and their digestion process takes 6 to 10 hours.

— Their colon is short and contains smooth alkaline.

Herbivore

— Examples of the Herbivore species include deer, buffaloes, giraffes, goats, sheep, etc.

— The psychological food of these animals includes grass and tree foliage.

— These animals walk on four paws with hooves, not claws.

— Their mouth opening is small and consists of the following teeth structure: rudimentary, blunt canines, big and flattened incisors and flattened, strong molars.

— Herbivore species cannot shear their food but they rather chew it a lot.

— They have big salivary glands and their alkaline saliva does contain ptyalin.

— These animals have a weak hydrochloric acid and they do require fiber to stimulate peristalsis.

— Herbivore species metabolize a small amount of vitamin A and cholesterol.

— Their sweat glands are structured throughout the whole body.

— The intestine of herbivore species is 30 times the length of their spine length.

— Their colon is long and contains complex acid.

— While their digestion process takes 24 to 48 hours, they can metabolize cellulose

Frugivore

— Examples of frugivore animals include chimpanzees, orangutans, giant pandas, etc.

— The psychological food of frugivore animals includes fruits, vegetables and nuts.

— These animals can walk both upwards and on four paws.

— Their mouth opening is small to medium with the teeth structure consisting of flattened molars, big and flattened incisors and canines developed for defense.

— Instead of shearing their food, these animals eat food by chewing it.

— They have big salivary glands and their alkaline saliva does contain ptyalin.

— With a weak hydrochloric acid, these animals require fiber to stimulate peristalsis.

— These animals can metabolize small amounts of cholesterol and vitamin A.

— The sweat glands are structured throughout the whole body

— The intestine of frugivore animals is 12 times their spine length.

— Colon is long and contains sacculated acid.

— Frugivore animals cannot metabolize cellulose and their digestion process takes 12 to 18 hours

As you can see from the numerous examples listed above, the human anatomy is much closer, if not the same, as the anatomy of the fruit eating species, while the anatomy of the omnivore, carnivore and herbivore species differs in significant ways. Thus, we can conclude that humans are best designed to eat fruits, vegetables and nuts of different kinds, for better health and a prolonged life.

Chapter 2: The Benefits of a Plant Based Diet

While there is no doubt that humans were meant to be eating fruits, vegetables and nuts from the beginning, a shift took place that introduced a large confusion, mixing humans with the omnivore species. Scientifically speaking, a plant based diet is much more beneficial and less harmful for humans, which is why it is recommended to shift from meat to whole grains, legumes, vegetables and other nutritional foods of this kind.

Switching to a plant based diet is beneficial for many reasons. If you're suffering from any kind of illnesses or have obesity issues, you should focus on a plant based diet as a way to better your health and reduce your symptoms, if not cure the illness completely. Nutrition is a powerful tool that can be used for great purposes, such as helping relieve pain and health problems, improving metabolism and the immune system, as well as strengthen your body and improve your mood.

Even if you don't have any health-related problems, you should transition to a plant based diet as a means of preventive health building. The natural ingredients such as fruits, beans or vegetables are full of nutritional values needed for the everyday functioning of our systems. In all cases, natural food is always better than processed food, as it doesn't contain any chemicals or unnatural substances that could be harmful to our health.

Besides boosting your health, a plant based diet can decrease the risks of many diseases, among them the most serious ones such as heart diseases, type 2 diabetes and certain types of cancers. Many studies at research facilities have proven these statements to be correct, such as, for example, a study conducted in JAMA Internal Medicine, which tracked over 70 000 people and their eating habits. This study has proven that a plant based diet can significantly improve your health and lengthen your life as well. Therefore, switching to a plant based diet is one of the best things you can do for yourself and your overall well-being.

People who consume plant based ingredients have a lower risk of developing diseases or having strokes because of the fibers, vitamins and minerals that come along with a plant based diet. These fibers, vitamins and minerals, as well as healthy fats, are essential substances your body needs in order to function properly. Plant based diets thus improve the blood lipid levels and better your brain health as well. There is a significant decrease in bad cholesterol in people who follow a plant based diet.

It is never too late to change your diet! Whether you're 18, 36 or 50, it is still recommended to switch to a plant based diet, as it is never too late to do so! These diets have quick and effective results that you will be noticing even after the first week of eating only plant-based meals. The first results you will notice will be the sense of accomplishment and satisfaction that comes with following a healthy diet. You will notice your mood has improved, in addition to not feel heavy after a meal, but instead feeling full and satisfied and yet energetic. After a period of following a plant-based diet, you will begin to notice the health benefits of doing so. Your health-related problems will be reduced and you will feel a significant relief in terms of pains or discomfort you've been having.

What is important to know when switching to a plant-based diet is that you are not going to be on any kind of deprivation diet. Many people relate plant based diets as diets where you are depriving yourself of meats and dairy foods. However, when you switch to a plant based diet you will not feel like you are missing anything, since your taste will adapt to your new eating habits. This will lead to you finding foods delicious that you probably disliked before. The human body is adapting constantly to the different inputs, and after a while, plant based foods will feel tasty and natural to you. The foods prepared of the healthy, nutritional ingredients are very delicious, especially if you follow the right recipes. Stick through this diet guide to learn some great plant based diet recipes you can include in your transition program. Once you see the benefits of the plant based diet and try some of the specialties, you will never want to go back to your eating habits again.

Transitioning from a meat to a plant based diet is not as difficult as everyone thinks. You can do it gradually, by increasing your fruit and vegetable intake while decreasing your meat and dairy intake. Minimizing meat consumption at first will make the transition seem effortless later, as you don't have to introduce drastic changes immediately. Instead of meat and dairy, you should start consuming the following foods:

— fruits such as apples, bananas, grapes, etc.

— vegetables such as kale, lettuce, peppers, corn, etc.

— tubers such as potatoes, beets, carrots, etc.

— whole grains such as rice, oats, millet, whole wheat, etc.

— legumes such as kidney beans, black beans, chickpeas, etc.

Therefore, your diet will be based on fruits, vegetables, tubers, whole grains and legumes. You can start implementing these changes by replacing meat in your favorite recipes and dishes with mushrooms or beans.

Gradually, you will completely lose the habit of consuming meat and switch to a full plant based diet. To help your transition process, you should add more calories of legumes, whole grains and vegetables to your everyday routine, as that will make you feel full and thus reduce your desire to eat meat and dairy.

As soon as you start switching your diet you will notice how positively your body reacts to receiving all the nutrients it needs to function properly. The foods you should be focusing on include beans, that is, all legumes, berries, broccoli, cabbage, collards, nuts and kale.

Before we get into the detailed, 4 week program for switching to a plant based diet, here are a few tips that will help you make the transition easily.

— Include fruits and vegetables in every meal of the day. Instead of snacking on chocolate bars, switch to fruit or nutritional bars. Remember, an apple a day keeps the doctor away!

— Downsize your meat servings gradually. Put less meat on your plate and more veggies. Make sure that the ¾ of the plate consists of plant-based ingredients!

You can slowly transition by introducing two or three meat-free days to your week plan. As time goes by you will get used to this system and you will be able to skip meat more often, until fully switching to the plant based diet.

Chapter 3: 4 Week Program for a Transition to a Plant Based Diet

In contrary to the popular belief, transitioning to a plant based diet is quite easy, if you take the right steps at the right time. By switching to a diet that includes more fibers, vitamins and minerals and avoiding meat and dairy products, you are not depriving yourself from any necessary nutrients. In fact, you are taking a step towards health improvement and a better life in general. Following this 4-week program for transitioning to a plant based diet will get you the results you wanted, which are healthy eating habits and the ability to enjoy food like you always did.

What is important to know when starting to transition to a plant based diet is that this process should be done gradually. You should by no means drop meat and dairy ingredients right away and strictly force yourself to eat plant based foods. The point of this program is to make your transition easy and effortless by gradually creating habits that are going to lead to a full transition without craving to return to your old eating habits. So, take it easy, step by step, and let's get into it!

Week 1

At the very beginning of your transition journey, you are going to start learning which foods to turn to and which ingredients to leave behind. The key here is to take things slowly, which is why in the first week you should focus on your breakfasts. Your meal plan for this week is going to consist of your regular meals with a bit of adjustments done to them. As this is the first stage of your plant based diet transition process, you need to start balancing your usual diet with the changes you are about to introduce to it. For the beginning, go through the contents of your refrigerator and try to take out as many animal products as possible. Stock your refrigerator with plant based ingredients to start your transition process! Foods you should be bringing into your fridge include berries, cabbage, broccoli, kale, beans, etc. Also, when choosing your ingredients, look for good quality and check the origin of the products, as you don't want anything processed to find a way to your kitchen.

Don't feel like you need to start avoiding meat and other animal foods right away. There should be no pressure to do so, as this is a calm and slow diet transition. In week 1 we are going to attack your breakfast habits while the rest of your meals of the day are going to stay the same. To help prepare yourself for the second week of your transition process, try to balance your plate by adding more plant based ingredients than you used to. The more you increase your whole foods intake at this stage of the transition, the easier it is going to be to adjust to what the second, third and fourth week has to offer! Therefore, in week 1, your goal is to switch to plant based breakfasts with fiber and high nutritional value. Here are three breakfast recipes for you to get inspired to start changing your morning meal habits.

#1 Three Minutes Oatmeal

Ingredients:

— 1/2 cup of oats

— 1 ripe banana

— 1 teaspoon of cinnamon

— 1 teaspoon of grounded flax seeds

— ½ cup of water

— ½ cup of plant based milk (soy/ rice/ almond/ hemp)

— Toppings of choice (peanut butter/ fresh fruit/ frozen berries/ seeds/ nuts)

Preparation:

Roast the oats, flax seeds together with cinnamon on a preheated non-stick pan for about 30 seconds. Add water and milk - start with little and rather add more to reach your desired consistency. Shortly before finishing, add sliced ripe banana (spotted), that is going to serve as a substitute for a sweetener.

Use this recipe as a base on how to prepare oatmeals and try to experiment with other ingredients such as frozen berries, nut butter, cacao, spices (turmeric), nuts or seeds. Mix those ingredients into the oatmeal either while cooking or only when serving as a topping.

Remember that you are trying to avoid processed foods. Therefore, do not forget to read the labels when purchasing your ingredients. Peanut butter should have only one ingredient - peanuts. You do not want any added salt, oil or sugar. The same is valid for dried fruits and plant based milk (avoid added sugar). It is simple, just read the ingredients of the products.

#2 Overnight Oats

Ingredients:

— ½ cup of oats

— ½ cup of nuts or seeds of choice (walnuts, hazelnuts, sunflower seeds, pumpkin seeds, ...)

— Dried fruit of choice (resins, cranberries, dates)

Preparation:

Do you want to prepare your breakfast the night before and not lose time in the morning? Just mix all the ingredients together and simply soak them overnight. In the morning just pour the excess water away and breakfast is served. If desired you can add some fresh fruit.

Soaking oats, nuts and seeds makes them easier digestible. It also wakes up a different taste in them, that you might have not experienced before.

#3 Green Smoothie

Smoothie is a go to breakfast when you want to start your day quickly and right away with a bunch of nutrients. The beauty of a smoothie is that you can add ingredients that you otherwise have problems adding to your diet. Perfect examples are greens such as spinach or kale.

For beginners, green smoothies might be quite a challenge. Therefore, I recommend starting with adding just a small portion of greens and slowly increase the amount over time as you get used to the taste.

Generally, the best basis for a smoothie are bananas as they make the smoothie nicely thick and naturally sweet. Always make sure that your fruits are ripe as fruit in that form is the easiest to digest. Ripe bananas are easy to recognize - the color is yellow (not green) with black spots.

Ingredients:

— 2 ripe bananas

— 1 cup fresh baby spinach

— 1 cup frozen berries

— 1 cup of water or plant based milk

Preparation:

First fill the blender with greens, then bananas or other fruits of your choice and liquid (water or plant based milk). Blend until smooth.

Week 2

In the second week of your transition to a plant based diet you should be used to eating whole foods and plant based ingredients for breakfast. Now we are going to step things up and introduce those ingredients to your lunch meals. Therefore, the second week of the program is going to consist of both breakfast and lunch meals made without animal products or any kinds of processed ingredients. You should focus on eliminating dairy products from your lunch meals as well as in general. There's no need to worry about calcium and other nutrients necessary for bone health, as you can get those from healthier plant based sources as well.

As the second week progresses, you will start learning how to effectively plan your meals and stay on track with your meal plans throughout the week. Dedicate a few minutes every Sunday to creating a meal plan for the following week. This way, you won't run out of ideas for breakfast, lunch or dinner for each day of the week. However, for now, we are only focusing on breakfast and lunch. Therefore, prepare to ditch animal food and combine plant-based ingredients into your lunch meals as well! Here are three recipes to get you started.

#1 Tortilla Pizza

Ingredients:

— Tortilla (optimally wholegrain)

— Tomato sauce or tomato paste

— Vegetable of choice as toppings (suggestion: sliced tomato, corn, garlic, red onion, ...)

— Herbs and spices (oregano, garlic powder)

— Nutritional yeast (optional)

Preparation:

Preheat your oven to 200°C.

If you are using bought tomato sauce then, as always, don't forget to check the ingredients. Make sure the sauce is not high in salt (the salt intake should not exceed 1 gram for 100 gram of the sauce) and that all ingredients are plant based: no cheese, meat or eggs.

If you decided to make your own sauce, also check the package of the tomato paste for the salt intake. Place the paste on a pan and add a little bit of water as the paste itself is thick already. When using this sauce for pizza I would recommend keeping it rather thicker. However, you can use the same sauce as a pasta sauce. In that case water it down. Add a teaspoon of dried oregano and a teaspoon of garlic powder. You might also want to add some chili if you prefer spicy food. If you want to add a bit of cheesy flavor to the sauce mix in also a tablespoon of nutritional yeast. You can also sprinkle the whole pizza with nutritional yeast once it is ready to be baked.

As your sauce is ready, spread it on a tortilla like you would do on a pizza dough. Now is the time to get creative with your favorite pizza toppings. If you want to top it with basil leaves or some greens, I recommend doing so only after the baking process as the leaves would burn in the oven.

To bake your pizza faster, and for more crunchy results, do not use baking tin and only bake the pizza on the grate.

Lower the temperature of the oven to 180°C and bake the pizza for approximately 15 minutes until the crust turns brown.

#2 Baked Sweet Potatoes with Avocado-Beans salad

Ingredients:

— 1 big or 2 small sweet potatoes

— ½ of an avocado

— ½ can of red beans

— 1 cup fresh spinach

— 1 tomato

— Pepper, salt (optional)

Preparation:

Preheat the oven to 250°C. Wash the sweet potatoes and poke a few holes in them using a knife to fasten the baking process. Place the potatoes on a baking paper in the oven, lower the temperature to 200°C and bake for about 40 to 60 minutes. The baking time is always dependent on your oven. Sweet potatoes are fully baked once sugar is running out of them and they are fork tender.

Meanwhile you have time to prepare your filling. Mash one half of an avocado in a bowl, add beans, diced tomato, pepper (freshly grounded if possible) and optionally salt and mix it all together. In general, try to slowly leave out salt from your diet - especially table salt. Don't worry; your taste buds quickly adapt to new tastes and you will not miss added salt in your meals after a short period of time. If you are not ready to leave out table salt out of your diet, substitute it rather with sea salt or pink Himalayan salt.

Once the potatoes are baked, cut them open. Mash the inside with a fork and create space for the filling. Add spinach leaves first and the avocado mixture on the top. Enjoy!

As with every dish in this book, try not to get stuck with a certain recipe. I would like to give you a guideline for the beginning. Moreover, I would like to encourage you to be creative. Nobody says you cannot add paprika next time instead of tomato, chickpeas instead of red beans or hummus instead of avocado. Remember you are adapting a new lifestyle, not just dieting for 4 weeks.

#3 Red Lentil Soup

Ingredients:

— 1 cup red lentils

— 4 cups of water or low- sodium veggie broth

— 1 table spoon olive oil

— 1 large carrot (diced)

— 1 large onion (diced)

— 1 ½ teaspoon of grounded cardamom

— ½ teaspoon of salt

— Black pepper

— Juice of 1 lemon

Preparation:

Heat olive oil in a big pot. Add onion and cardamom, salt and little bit of black pepper and stir until the onion turns little brown. Add lentils and carrots and stir to combine. In this time, the soup is getting its most flavor, so spend a few minutes constantly mixing it, so it doesn't burn at the bottom.

Finally add water or veggie broth (4 cups for each cup of lentils), cover the pot and let it cook on low heat for about 15- 20 minutes.

How do you recognize if it's done? Firstly, when tasting the lentils. Red lentils are falling apart while cooking. Therefore they should be melting in your mouth when tasting. Secondly, check the carrots with stabbing a piece with a knife. Once the piece slides down the knife, the carrot is cooked. In case it sticks on the knife, keep cooking. This rule generally counts for coking any kind of root vegetable.

When finished cooking, add freshly squeezed lemon juice. Mix it all in and enjoy.

You can keep the soup refrigerated for 5 days. However, it is going to thicken with every day, so you can either water it down or keep it as it is and use it as sauce to be eaten with rice, couscous, quinoa or bread.

Week 3

In week three you are going to switch your dinner meals to the plant based diet, that is, use only plant based ingredients to prepare your food. With the third week, you are already wrapping up the transition, as you are now used to your new breakfast and lunch meal strategies. All it takes now is to start implementing those strategies to your dinner meals. At this point, you should already be feeling the improvement in your life caused by starting to transition to a plant based diet.

With numerous recipes and tips, making plant based meals is quick and easy, yet as delicious and healthy as you can imagine! In your week three of the transition process you are already near the end of it. What's left to do is introduce these change to your dinner meals as well and in that way, wrap up a completely new meal plan you are going to be creating every Sunday to stay on track with what you're eating! Here are some delicious and easy plant based dinner recipes!

#1 Bulgur Salad

Ingredients:

— ½ cup bulgur wheat

— Diced vegetable of your choice (paprika, celery, tomatoes)

— ½ cup chickpeas

— 1 cup spinach (diced)

— ½ avocado

— Pepper, salt, oregano, powdered garlic

Preparation:

There are two options how to prepare bulgur. If you need to prepare your dish quickly, then simply cook bulgur (1 cup bulgur for 2 cups cold water) in a pot. Bring to a boil, cover the pot and let simmer for 12-15 minutes until tender.

Another option is to soak the bulgur before. Ideally, overnight, but already an hour is enough. Strain it afterwards, rinse one more time and you're good to go. The soaked version tastes lighter and refreshing.

Mash an avocado in a bowl and combine with bulgur. Add in chickpeas and prepared vegetables diced on small pieces. Finally add in seasonings according to your taste. Give it a final mix and enjoy!

#2 Almond noodles

Ingredients:

— 100 g of whole grain spaghetti

— ½ cup of almond butter

— ¼ cup of water

— ¼ cup of rice vinegar

— 2 tablespoons of low sodium soy sauce or tamari

— 2 tablespoons of Thai red curry paste

— Chopped fresh cilantro

Preparation:

To prepare this nutrient rich and flavorful dish, cook the spaghetti as you regularly would, while, in the meantime, mix the almond butter, rice vinegar, water, soy sauce or tamari and the Thai red curry paste and whisk it together in a large bowl. Once the spaghetti is cooked, add it into the sauce and mix it together. Serve the meal with the chopped cilantro on top and enjoy!

#3 Pumpkin Soup

Ingredients:

— 500 g pumpkin (without seeds)

— 3 cloves garlic (unpeeled)

— 1 table spoon olive oil

— Pepper (amount depending on your own taste)

— ½ teaspoon Turmeric

— Salt (optional)

— Cayenne pepper, chilli (optional)

— Boiled water or low- sodium veggie broth

Preparation:

Preheat your oven to 200°C.

Remove the pumpkin seeds and cut the pumpkin to pieces about 2 inches big. Mix them in a bowl together with garlic cloves, olive oil, pepper, turmeric, salt if needed and if you like spicy food you can also add cayenne pepper or chilli powder.

Spread prepared pumpkin on a baking tin with baking sheet (moisturize the baking tin, so the baking sheet sticks on it), place the tin in the oven. Lover its temperature to 180°C and bake for about 40 minutes. Once done, the pumpkin will be fork tender.

Finally place the mixture in a blender (or pot when using submersible blender). Do not forget to free the garlic cloves from its peel. Add two cups of boiled water or veggie broth and blend it all together. Keep adding liquid to achieve the desired thickness of your soup.

Finally, you can always add more spices or salt, if you feel like the soup still needs more taste.

To mix up the recipe, replace the pumpkin with carrots or sweet potatoes. As always, be creative and have fun!

Week 4

In the final stage of the transition process you should already be used to the new eating habits you've developed. You have switched your breakfast, lunch and dinner meals to plant based meals but the journey doesn't end there! You still have got a lot to learn, from how to combat cravings to how to make some of the most delicious plant based meals ever! To combat your cravings, increase the intake of plant based ingredients per meal to feel fuller and less prone to satisfy a craving.

Throughout the fourth week of the program and after, you are going to be learning about new recipes that involve great plant based meals. Learning new recipes is going to help you keep your meal plan diverse and full of nutrients. Your plant based diet adventure does not end with this program! After the fourth week, you will be used to this type of diet but you will still have a lot to learn and a lot of material to experiment with. One very important thing to learn at this stage of the program is that you should be eating plant based, healthy snacks every day to feel fuller and reduce cravings, as well as stay energetic and productive throughout the day. Stay consistent with your meal plans and include snacks every now and then. Of course, the easiest and always go to snack should be fruit and vegetables or nuts. There is nothing easier than pull out an apple or few nuts from your bag when on the go. To make your transition smoother, make always sure you have a little snack always with you, so you don't end up eating fast food or some other processed foods. Remember you came to this world with only one body and you are not getting any other. So, you better take good care of it.

Did you have fun in the kitchen last three weeks and you feel like discovering more fun recipes, that can make your snacks more diverse and creative? Here are three great recipes for plant-based snacks!

#1 Two-Ingredients Banana- Oatmeal cookies

Ingredients:

— 1 large ripe banana

— 1 cup oats

Preparation:

Simply mash the banana and mix in the oats. If desired you can still add one of following ingredients (raisins, dried cranberries, cocoa nibs, shredded coconut, chopped nuts).

Shape tablespoons of dough on a baking sheet in a form of cookies. Bake in the oven heated on 180°C for about 10 minutes. Let them cool after taking out of the oven and enjoy.

#2 Coconut Bites

Ingredients:

— 1 cup of pineapple juice

— 2 cups of diced mango

— 2 diced ripe bananas

— ½ vanilla bean

— 4 cups of shredded coconut

— ¾ cup of toasted shredded coconut

Preparation:

Use a small pot to cook the pineapple juice, bananas, mango and vanilla. Cook at low heat for five minutes. Then scrape the seeds from the vanilla bean into the pot and cook for two more minutes. Put the ingredients into the pot, process the 4 cups of shredded coconut until you have a smooth but firm mixture. Let the mixture cool down for an hour or two and then a roll small amount of it into a ball and roll it into the toasted coconut. Roll up all your coconut bites for a perfect plant based snack!

#3 Fruit Pie

Ingredients:

— 1 cup of pitted dates

— 1 ½ cup of walnuts or pecans

— 1 tablespoon of vanilla extract

— ½ cup of shredded coconut

— ½ tablespoon of cinnamon

— Sliced fresh fruit

Preparation:

Put all crust ingredients into a food processor and blend them until you get a paste. Press the paste into a pie pan and let it chill for a while, until it is ready to add fruit on it. Arrange the fruit on top of the pie according to your liking and cool the pie off 1 hour before serving and, voila, a perfect, healthy snack.

Summary

This plant-based diet guide was designed to introduce beginners to this kind of diet and encourage them to make the right choices regarding their eating habits. As a beginner, you don't have to feel overwhelmed and pressured by diet plans. Instead of jumping straight into it, it is more important to firstly get to know the diet and learn why it is beneficial for your health and overall well-being. That's exactly what this book was designed to do, teach you about the plant-based diet and show you how to gradually yet surly transition to a diet without any animal products. What you should take away from this book are all the reasons why the plant-based diet positively affects your health and why it is important to manage your eating habits regularly. Upon getting to know all this information, the next step is to start implementing it in your everyday life. Ditching animal products completely sounds like a difficult task but it can actually be easy and effortless, as long as you follow the right meal plan. My plant-based diet guide will help you effortlessly transition to a plant-based diet by introducing new ingredients gradually, without pressure. Throughout this 4 week program, you will get used to plant-based ingredients and start letting go of animal products up until the point where you completely throw them out of your everyday meals. Keep in mind that diet transition is a steady process, so don't try to rush and skip steps of the meal program in hopes to achieve the results sooner. Take it easy and enjoy combining various delicious ingredients and preparing outstanding meals while receiving all the necessary nutrients for your body's proper functioning.

Conclusion

Thank you again for purchasing this book!

I hope this book was able to help you easily transition to a plant based diet and gain all its health benefits!

The next step is to start enjoying your new meal plans and keep learning about new and delicious recipes!

Finally, if you enjoyed this book, then I would like to ask you for a favor, would you be kind enough to leave a review for this book on Amazon? It would be greatly appreciated!

Thank you and good luck!

Made in the USA
San Bernardino, CA
24 May 2018